THE NEW ILEOSTOMY DIET COOKBOOK FOR BEGINNERS

Deliciously Simple Recipes to Prevent Stoma Blockage, Heal Your Bowel, and Improve Digestive Health

Michael Slowick, RDN

COPYRIGHT PAGE

to ensure the accuracy of the information provided herein, no promises are made regarding its completeness or accuracy. Any statements made by sales employees or representatives, whether verbal or written, do not constitute extended or implied guarantees.

Table of Contents

CHAPTER I: INTRODUCTION TO ILEOSTOMY

An ileostomy is an opening in the belly (abdominal wall) that's made during surgery. It's usually needed because a problem is causing the ileum to not work properly, or a disease is affecting that part of the colon and it needs to be removed. The end of the ileum (the lowest part of the small intestine) is brought through this opening to form a stoma, usually on the lower right side of the abdomen. An ileostomy may only be needed for a short time (temporary), maybe for 3 to 6 months, because that part of the colon needs time to rest and heal from a problem or disease. But sometimes a disease, such as cancer, is more serious and an ileostomy may be needed for the rest of a person's life (permanent).

A Wound Ostomy Continence nurse (WOCN or WOC nurse) will probably work with the surgeon to figure out the best location and way to care for your stoma. (A WOC nurse is a specially trained registered nurse who takes care of and teaches ostomy patients. This nurse may also be called an ostomy nurse.)

When you look at your stoma, you are actually looking at the lining (the mucosa) of your small intestine, which looks a lot like the inside lining of your cheek. The stoma will look pink to red. It's warm and moist and secretes small amounts of mucus. It will shrink shortly after surgery. Its shape will be round to oval. Some stomas may stick out a little, while others are flat against the skin.

Unlike the anus, the stoma has no valve or shut-off muscle. This means you won't be able to control stool passing from the stoma. There are no nerve endings in the stoma, so the stoma itself is not a source of pain or discomfort.

As part of this surgery, the colon (the main part of large intestine) and rectum (the lowest part of large intestine where formed stool is held until it's passed out of the body through the anus) are often removed (this is called a colectomy). This means that colon and rectum no longer function as they used to. Sometimes, only part of the colon and rectum are removed.

What does an ileostomy do?

After the colon and rectum are removed or bypassed, waste no longer comes out of the body through the rectum and anus. Digestive contents now leave the body through the stoma. The drainage is collected in a pouch that sticks to the skin around the stoma. The pouch is fitted to you personally. It's worn at all times and can be emptied as needed.

Ileostomy output will be liquid to pasty, depending on what you eat, your medicines, and other factors. Because the output is constant, you'll need to empty the pouch 5 to 8 times a day.

Categories of ileostomy

There are two main categories of ileostomy: end and loop. Both ileostomies work similarly. You won't have control of when poop comes out of the ostomy into the bag, so you'll need to wear your bag all the time. Some ileostomies are reversible, and some are permanent.

Loop ileostomy

Your surgeon will do a loop ileostomy when there's a connection of the intestine with the colon that needs to be protected. In that case, the surgeon goes "upstream" of the connection and brings up a loop of small intestine (the ileum) through the hole in your abdominal wall. Then, they'll open a part of your intestine and sew it to your skin so poop can exit into an ostomy bag.

End ileostomy

During an end ileostomy, a surgeon will bring the very end of your small intestine through your abdominal wall.

Types of Ileostomy

An ileostomy can be permanent, or it might be reversed after the condition for which it was needed has healed. In still another circumstance, the ileostomy is used as a step between other surgeries.

An ileostomy is not a colostomy. With a colostomy, part of the large intestine is used to make the stoma.

Permanent Ileostomy

In a permanent ileostomy, the end of the small intestine is brought through the abdomen to create a stoma. This might also be called an end ileostomy or a Brooke ileostomy.

After food is eaten, it travels down the esophagus, into the stomach, through the small intestine, and out of the body through the stoma. It is collected in a bag (sometimes also called a pouch) worn over the stoma. The stool tends to be looser than it was before the surgery. The stoma bag is emptied several times a day.

The ileostomy is permanent when there is no plan or ability to reverse it. The colon, rectum, and/or anus may have been removed or there may be a plan to remove them in the future. Or, there is no possibility of those areas healing.

Temporary Ileostomy

A temporary ileostomy is reversible. That means the stoma will be removed, and the person will eliminate waste the way they had presurgery.

A temporary ostomy may also be called a diverting ostomy. The stoma is not formed from the end of the small intestine. But rather, thinking of the small intestine like a tube, it is cut almost in half and bent back on itself.

There are two openings, one that allows stool to leave the body. The other opening allows for the drainage of any mucus created by the part of the digestive system not used for stool.

Reasons for Ileostomy Surgery

If you have a large intestine problem that can't be treated with medications, you might need an ileostomy. One of the most common reasons for an ileostomy is inflammatory bowel disease (IBD). The two types of inflammatory bowel disease are **Crohn's disease** and **ulcerative colitis.**

Crohn's disease can involve any part of the digestive tract, from the mouth to the anus, causing inflammation of the lining with sores and scarring.

Ulcerative colitis also has inflammation, sores, and scarring but involves the large intestine and rectum.

People with IBD will often find blood and mucus in their stool, and experience weight loss, poor nutrition, and abdominal pain.

Other problems that might require an ileostomy include:

Rectal or colon cancer

An inherited condition called familial polyposis, in which polyps form in the colon that can lead to cancer

Intestinal birth defects

Injuries or accidents that involve the intestines

Hirschsprung's disease

Procedure and Recovery

An ileostomy is done in a hospital under general anesthesia.

After you're unconscious, your surgeon will either make a cut down your midline or perform a laparoscopic procedure using smaller cuts and lighted instruments. You will know prior to the surgery which method is recommended for your condition. Depending on your condition, your surgeon may need to remove your rectum and colon.

There are several different types of permanent ileostomies.

For a standard ileostomy, the surgeon makes a small incision that will be the site of your ileostomy. They'll pull a loop of your ileum through the incision. This part of your intestine is turned inside out, exposing the inner surface. It's soft and pink, like the inside of a cheek. The part that sticks out is called a stoma. It may protrude up to 2 inches.

People with this type of ileostomy, also called a Brooke ileostomy, won't have control of when their fecal waste flows into the external plastic pouch.

Another type of ileostomy is the continent, or Kock, ileostomy. Your surgeon uses part of your small intestine to form an internal pouch with an external stoma that serves as a valve. These are stitched to your abdominal wall. A few times per day you insert a flexible tube through the stoma and into the pouch. You expel your waste through this tube.

The advantages of the Kock ileostomy are that there's no external pouch and you can control when you empty your waste. This procedure is known as a K-pouch procedure. It's often the preferred method of ileostomy because it eliminates the need for an external pouch.

A different procedure, known as the J-pouch procedure, may be performed if you've had your entire colon and rectum removed. In this procedure, the doctor creates an internal pouch from the ileum that is then connected to the anal canal, allowing you to expel your waste through the usual route with no need for a stoma.

Recovery from ileostomy

You'll typically need to stay in the hospital for at least three days. It's not uncommon to remain hospitalized for a week or even longer, especially if your ileostomy was done under emergency circumstances.

Your food and water intake will be limited for a while. On the day of your surgery, you may only get ice chips. Clear liquids will probably be allowed on the second day. Slowly, you'll be able to eat more solid foods as your bowels adjust to the changes.

In the early days after surgery, you may have excessive intestinal gas. This will decrease as your intestines heal. Some people have found that digesting four to five small meals per day is better than three larger meals. Your doctor may suggest that you avoid certain foods for a while.

During your recovery, whether you have an internal or external pouch, you'll start to learn how to manage the pouch that will collect your waste. You'll also learn to care for your stoma and the skin around it. Enzymes in the discharge from your ileostomy can irritate your skin. You'll need to keep the stoma area clean and dry.

If you have an ileostomy, you may find that you need to make big adjustments to your lifestyle. Some people seek help from an ostomy support group. Meeting other people who've adjusted their lifestyles after this surgery and have managed to return to their regular activities can ease any anxieties you have.

You can also find nurses who are specially trained in ileostomy management. They'll ensure that you have a manageable lifestyle with your ileostomy.

Ileostomy Risks and Complications

Having surgery will come with some risks. The surgical team will review these risks during the pre-op appointments and answer any questions. Some general risks of most surgeries include anesthetic complications, bleeding, blood clots, delayed healing, difficulty breathing, infection, injury, or poor results.

Certain complications are specific to ileostomy procedures. Some of the potential problems that can occur after getting a stoma include:

Peristomal dermatitis: The area around the stoma is called the peristomal skin. The ileostomy output, which can be watery and contain irritating substances, may cause the skin to break down.

Ischemia/necrosis: It is not common, but the tissue can start to die when the blood flow to the stoma is cut off for some reason. The stoma may become dark and swollen. Depending on the situation's seriousness, emergency surgery may be needed to reconstruct the stoma.

Retraction: A stoma could potentially go back under the skin and sit flush with the abdominal wall. This can make fitting an ostomy pouch difficult. Products called convex appliances may help. However, some people may need to find another solution, which could mean revision surgery.

Small bowel obstruction: Surgery on the bowels has a risk of causing an obstruction (blockage). Depending on the severity of the blockage, home remedies may clear it, but it could also be treated in the hospital with decompression. Uncommonly, more surgery might be needed.

High-output stoma: Some people find that their stoma has a lot of output (the term for stool from an ostomy). This can lead to fatigue and dehydration. Sometimes, antidiarrheal drugs may be used to slow it down. People with a high-output stoma will also want to talk about replacing fluids with their healthcare team, either by drinking or with an intravenous (IV) line.

Stomal prolapse: A prolapse is when the stoma extends outward too far. It can be painful. Sometimes, the stoma can be pushed back in (reduced) by hand by a healthcare provider or by applying a sugar solution to it.

Parastomal hernia: A hernia can form near the stoma. A hernia is when the intestines protrude into a weak spot in the abdominal wall. It can be painful and make it difficult to attach the pouching system to the abdomen.

Long-term outlook

Once you learn to take care of your new elimination system, you'll be able to participate in most of your regular activities. People with ileostomies:

swim

hike

play sports

eat in restaurants

camp

travel

work in most occupations

Heavy lifting can be a problem because it can aggravate your ileostomy. Talk to your doctor if your job requires heavy lifting.

Having an ileostomy doesn't usually interfere with sexual function or the ability to have children. It might require you to educate your sexual partners, who might be unfamiliar with ileostomies. You should discuss your ostomy with your partner before progressing to intimacy.

CHAPTER II: BASICS OF ILEOSTOMY DIET

It's best to eat mostly bland, low-fiber foods for the first few weeks after your surgery. Bland foods are cooked, easy-to-digest foods that aren't spicy, heavy, or fried. Eating bland foods will help you avoid uncomfortable symptoms, such as:

• Diarrhea (loose or watery bowel movements)

• Bloating

• Gas

• Swelling or tenderness at your ileostomy site

General Eating and Drinking Guidelines

Follow these guidelines for the first few weeks after your surgery. This will help keep you comfortable while your colon heals.

Eat small meals often.

Try to have 6 small meals throughout the day instead of 3 large ones.

Don't eat too much in the evening. This will help limit the bowel movements (poop) from your ileostomy during the night.

Drink 8 to 10 (8-ounce) glasses (about 2 liters) of liquids every day. This will help you replace the water lost through your ileostomy and keep you from becoming dehydrated (losing more fluid from your body than usual).

Eat mostly bland, low-fiber foods.

When you add foods back into your diet, introduce them 1 at a time.

Before you're discharged (released) from the hospital, a clinical dietitian nutritionist will talk with you about these guidelines. After you leave the hospital, your doctor and an outpatient clinical dietitian nutritionist will help you as you go back to following your usual diet.

Eat slowly and chew your food well to help with digestion.

Importance of Diet Post-Ileostomy Surgery

After ileostomy surgery, paying attention to your diet is crucial. Here's why:

Nutrient Absorption: Your body may have difficulty absorbing certain nutrients, like vitamins A, D, E, K, and electrolytes such as potassium and magnesium. A balanced diet ensures you're getting what you need.

Hydration: Dehydration can be a risk due to increased fluid losses. Drinking enough fluids is vital for your overall health and to prevent complications.

Avoiding Bowel Issues: Some foods, especially high-fiber ones, might cause bowel blockages or worsen diarrhea. Knowing what to eat can prevent discomfort and complications.

Managing Output: Certain foods can affect the consistency and frequency of output from the stoma. Adjusting your diet can help control these factors.

Promoting Healing: A nutritious diet supports tissue repair and wound healing, essential for recovery after surgery.

Overall Health: Eating well doesn't just address nutritional needs; it supports your overall well-being, energy levels, and immune function.

Lifestyle Adjustment: Life with an ileostomy often means changing your eating habits. Working with healthcare professionals can help you navigate these changes and lead a fulfilling life.

In summary, your diet post-ileostomy surgery is vital for your recovery, health, and adjustment to your new normal. Working with healthcare professionals can guide you in making the best choices for your well-being.

Key Nutrients and Their Importance

• Include protein foods such as meat, fish, eggs, cheese and milk to help with wound healing

• Eat starchy carbohydrates such as white bread, low fibre cereals (rice krispies, cornflakes), potato (no skin), white rice/pasta, for energy and to thicken your stoma output

- If your appetite is low, try taking smaller meals and snacks in between such as a small bowl of cereal, sandwich, cheese and crackers, yogurts or milky drinks.

Preventing Dehydration

When you have an ileostomy, you lose much more salt, potassium, and water than usual. This can lead to dehydration.

Throughout each day, keep track of your liquid intake (how much liquid you drink). You should also keep track of your ostomy output (how much liquid comes out of your ileostomy). Record your liquid intake and ostomy output. Your nurse will give you a measuring cup before you leave the hospital.

Call your doctor's office if your output is more than 1000 milliliters (about 34 ounces) per day or is watery. They may recommend a fiber supplement or medication.

Signs of dehydration

Being dehydrated, even for less than 24 hours, can lead to kidney failure. Kidney failure happens when your kidneys can't do their normal functions.

Dizziness

Dark, amber-colored urine (pee)

Headaches

Muscle cramps

Dry mouth or cracked lips

Urinating (peeing) less than usual

Feeling more thirsty than usual

Heart palpitations (an unusually fast, strong, or irregular heartbeat)

Loss of appetite (not feeling hungry)

Emptying your pouch more than usual (such as every hour).

Guidelines for preventing dehydration

Follow these guidelines to help keep you from becoming dehydrated.

Aim to drink 8 to 10 (8-ounce) glasses (about 2 liters) of liquids every day.

Don't drink more than 4 ounces (½ cup) of liquids with meals. Don't drink any liquids for 1 hour before and 1 hour after meals. This helps make your bowel movements bulkier.

It's important to keep drinking lots of liquids, even if your bowel movements are watery. Drinking less liquid won't help your bowel movements be less watery, and it can lead to dehydration.

Drink sports drinks (such as Gatorade or Powerade) and oral rehydration solutions (such as Pedialyte). These drinks will help replace your fluid loss quickly, especially if your ostomy output is high. A high output is more than 1000 milliliters (about 34 ounces) per day. If you don't have these drinks, you can make your own using these ingredients:

4 cups (32 ounces, which is about 1 liter) of water

1 cup (8 ounces) of orange juice

8 teaspoons (40 milliliters) of sugar

1 teaspoon (4 milliliters) of salt

Put all ingredients into a cup with a lid. Shake well so the sugar and salt dissolve (melt).

Limit or avoid the following foods and drinks. They can cause diarrhea or watery bowel movements, which makes you more likely to become dehydrated.

Limit liquids with caffeine (such as caffeinated tea and coffee) and liquids high in fat (such as regular milk) to 1 cup (8 ounces) per day.

If you drink coffee, choose a dark roast instead of a light roast. Dark roast coffee usually has less caffeine than light roast coffee because some caffeine is lost during the roasting process.

Limit the amount of alcohol you drink for the first 3 weeks after your surgery. Alcohol can cause you to lose more fluid. Talk with your healthcare provider for more information.

Don't drink sugary drinks, such as juice and soda. If you want to drink juice, choose 100% fruit juice and dilute it (mix it with water) to reduce the sugar. To do this, add 1 part water to 1 part of juice (for example, 4 ounces of water mixed with 4 ounces of juice).

Don't have artificial sweeteners, such as sorbitol, mannitol, and xylitol. Artificial sweeteners are often found in sugar-free drinks, candies, gum, and cough drops.

Eat foods that contain electrolytes. Electrolytes, such as sodium and potassium, can help prevent dehydration. The following table includes examples of foods that are high in sodium and potassium.

Foods high in sodium

Broth

Buttermilk

Cheese

Commercially prepared or processed packaged foods (such as TV dinners)

Puréed canned soups (smooth and easy to swallow)

Salted pretzels

Saltine crackers

Soy sauce

Table salt

Tomato juice

Bananas

Don't eat more than 1 small ripe banana per day for the first 3 to 4 weeks after your surgery. Eating more than this may cause an ileostomy blockage.

Foods high in potassium

Broccoli

Coconut water

Chicken, fish, and veal

Orange juice without pulp

Oranges without seeds or membrane (the thin clear or white part around each section)

Potatoes without the skin

Soy milk

Tomato or vegetable soup

Turkey

Yogurt

CHAPTER III: OVERVIEW OF DIGESTIVE CHANGES

In first few days Your surgeon will suggest you start with free fluids and move to a soft, moist, low fibre diet.

Initially you may find fibrous foods are difficult to digest and may cause a blockage if they are eaten in large quantities or not properly chewed. Therefore, it is advised to avoid these at this time. Foods that are high in insoluble fibre and you may wish to avoid at first include:

Celery

Coconut

Fruit – especially dried fruit, pith and skin

Lettuce

Mango

Mushrooms

Nuts

Pineapple

Pips

Seeds

Sweetcorn

Vegetables – skin on

The small bowel will slowly adapt, and the output should decrease. The introduction of solid, low fibre food helps the small bowel to begin to work as normal and allows the stool to thicken and become less watery. The stool you pass into your bag will thicken to a 'porridge-like' consistency and the bag will need to be emptied less. Your output should settle around 6-8 weeks.

2 months after Surgery

Within 6-8 weeks post-surgery, the remaining small bowel usually adapts, and the stoma output usually decreases to around 800ml per day. The aim is for a 'porridge-like' consistency. At this point you can start to gradually include foods higher in fibre again and reduce salt intake. Once the stoma output has decreased you can return to a normal diet and focus on healthy eating rather than eating for your ileostomy bag.

Low Appetite

It may take time for your appetite to return to normal after surgery. Until you are able to manage normal quantities of food again eat 'little and often'. Aim to eat small meals and snacks every 2-3 hours. These could consist of smaller meals with snacks, such as cereal, sandwiches, yoghurts, cheese and crackers and nutritious drinks like milk, shop bought or homemade milkshakes. Aim for small portions of high energy foods. Eating regularly during the daytime also helps your ileostomy output, whereas late evening meals may increase ileostomy output during the night. You could try increasing your intake in the day and having only a small meal in the evening. If your appetite continues to be poor and/or you are losing weight please contact your healthcare professional or stoma

nurse as soon as possible.

Healthy Eating with an Established Ileostomy

There is no long-term specific diet for a person with an ileostomy. Healthy eating is important for your general well-being. Try not to restrict your diet unnecessarily. However, if you are experiencing specific problems contact your health professionals or stoma nurse.

Guidelines for Managing Common Problems

You don't need to follow these guidelines unless you're having the problems listed.

If certain foods caused discomfort before your surgery, they'll still cause discomfort after your surgery.

Diarrhea

Diarrhea is having loose or watery bowel movements, having more bowel movements than what's normal for you, or both. Diarrhea can be caused by:

Certain foods

Skipping meals

Food poisoning

An infection in your intestine

Antibiotics (medicines to treat infections) and other prescription medications

A blockage in your intestine

If you're having diarrhea, follow these guidelines:

Call your doctor's office. They may give you a medication to help.

Drink 8 to 10 (8-ounce) glasses (about 2 liters) of liquids throughout the day. Drink sports drinks (such as Gatorade or Powerade) and oral rehydration solutions (such as Pedialyte), if you can.

Don't eat the following foods and drinks. They may cause diarrhea. Foods that may cause diarrhea

Alcohol (such as beer and wine)

Bran

Broccoli

Brussels sprouts

Cabbage

Caffeinated drinks, especially hot drinks

Chocolate

Corn

Foods with artificial sweeteners (such as mannitol, sorbitol, and xylitol)

Fried meats, fish, and poultry

Fruit juice (such as prune, apple, grape, and orange juices)

Green leafy vegetables

High-fat foods

High-sugar foods

Legumes (such as cooked or dried beans)

Licorice

Milk and dairy products with lactose, if you're lactose intolerant

Nuts and seeds

Peas

Spicy foods

Stone fruits (such as apricots, peaches, plums, and prunes)

"Sugar-free" canned or dried fruits

Tomatoes

Turnip greens

Whole grains (such as wheat bread).

Eat more of the following foods. They may help thicken your bowel movements.

Foods that may help thicken bowel movements:

Applesauce

Bananas

Barley*

Boiled white rice

Cheese

Creamy nut butters (such as peanut butter)

Marshmallows

Oatmeal Pasta *

Potatoes without the skin

Pretzels

Saltine crackers

Tapioca

White bread

Yogurt

* These foods are whole grains. You can eat them if you're having diarrhea because they may help thicken your bowel movements.

Constipation

Constipation is having fewer than 3 bowel movements per week, having hard bowel movements, having a hard time passing bowel movements, or all 3. Constipation can be caused by:

Certain pain medications

Certain anti-nausea medications

Not eating enough fiber

Not exercising enough

Not drinking enough liquids

If you're constipated, follow these guidelines:

Call your doctor's office. They may give you a medication to help.

Drink hot water with lemon or lemon juice, coffee, or prune juice.

Do light exercise (such as walking), if you can.

Ask your doctor if eating high-fiber foods or taking a fiber supplement will help.

Gas and odor

For the first few weeks after your surgery, it's common to have gas in your pouch and a bad odor when you open your pouch. You may have more gas if you had a robotic surgery.

If you're having problems with gas or odor, talk with your wound, ostomy, and continence (WOC) nurse. You can also follow these guidelines:

Don't do these things. They can cause gas.

Chewing gum

Drinking with a straw

Smoking or chewing tobacco

Eating too fast

Skipping meals

Ask your healthcare provider if you can take an over-the-counter medication (such as Beano® or simethicone) before meals to help prevent gas.

Eat less of the following foods. They may cause gas, bad odor, or both. Foods that may cause gas, bad odor, or both

Asparagus

Alcohol, especially beer

Broccoli

Brussels sprouts

Cabbage

Carbonated drinks (such as soda)

Cauliflower

Corn

Dried beans and peas

Eggs

Fish

Garlic

Grapes

Leeks

Milk and dairy products with lactose, if you're lactose intolerant

Onions

Peanuts

Prunes

Eat more of the following foods. They may help prevent gas, bad odor, or both. Foods that may prevent gas, bad odor, or both

Buttermilk

Cranberry juice

Kefir

Parsley

Yogurt.

Managing Fiber Intake

What is fibre and why is it important?

 Fibre is found in plant-based foods and it increases the natural action of the gut bacteria, helping to form stools and regulate bowel opening. There are two main kinds of fibre; soluble and insoluble. Aim to include both types of fibre in your diet and drink plenty of fluids alongside fibrous foods to avoid constipation.

Soluble - as the name suggests dissolves in water and can help your stool soften. This can help with constipation and also help thicken your stool if your output is loose. Soluble fibre helps to lower cholesterol and regulates sugar in the blood. Soluble fibre is found in food such as the fleshy part of fruits and vegetables, oats, beans, peas, lentils and pulses. Insoluble - adds bulk, but doesn't dissolve in water, so will not break down as it passes through your digestive system. This type of fibre acts like a sponge in the digestive system and soaks up the moisture to form soft stools which are easily passed. However, if taken in amounts that are too high it might not be well tolerated, leading to bloating, wind and discomfort. Try small amounts at first, increasing depending on the effect on your output. Insoluble fibre is found in wholegrain and whole-meal flour, breads, pasta, rice, cereals, fruit and vegetable skins.

Insoluble - adds bulk, but doesn't dissolve in water, so will not break down as it passes through your digestive system. This type of fibre acts like a sponge in the digestive system and soaks up the moisture to form soft stools which are easily passed. However, if taken in amounts that are too high it might not be well tolerated, leading to bloating, wind and discomfort. Try small amounts at first, increasing depending on the effect on your output. Insoluble fibre is found in wholegrain and wholemeal flour, breads, pasta, rice, cereals, fruit and vegetable skins.

CHAPTER IV: NUTRITIONAL TIPS FOR ILEOSTOMY MANAGEMENT

When managing an ileostomy diet, it's crucial to prioritize foods that are gentle on digestion, won't lead to blockages, and assist in regulating stool consistency. Usually you should:

Opt for easily digestible fruits like bananas, peeled apples, ripe melons, and canned fruits without skins or seeds.

Cooked vegetables, such as carrots, spinach, green beans, and potatoes without skin, are easier on the digestive system.

Choose white bread, white rice, pasta, and refined cereals over whole grains to keep fiber intake low.

Incorporate lean protein sources like skinless poultry, fish, eggs, and tofu into your meals.

Dairy products can be included if well-tolerated; consider lactose-free options if lactose intolerance is a concern.

Smooth nut butters like peanut butter or almond butter offer protein and healthy fats without extra fiber.

Prefer refined grains such as white rice, white pasta, and couscous over whole grains.

Use small amounts of healthy fats like olive oil, canola oil, and butter for cooking or flavoring.

Smooth sauces and gravies can enhance flavor and moisture without adding bulk or fiber.

Indulge in soft desserts like gelatin, pudding, custard, and ice cream in moderation.

Foods to Avoid

In an ileostomy-friendly diet, it's wise to avoid foods that might lead to blockages, upset your digestive system, or cause discomfort. Foods to avoid include the following:

High-fiber foods: These include whole grains like whole wheat bread, brown rice, and whole grain cereals, as well as fibrous fruits and vegetables such as raw broccoli, cabbage, corn, and berries.

Tough meats: Steer clear of meats that are difficult to chew or digest, such as tough cuts of beef or pork, and meats with gristle or skin.

Nuts and seeds: These can be hard to digest and may cause blockages in your digestive system. Avoid whole nuts, seeds, and foods containing them, like granola or trail mix.

Stringy vegetables: Vegetables with tough or stringy fibers, like celery and asparagus, can be challenging for your digestive system to process.

Dried fruits: Dried fruits, such as raisins, prunes, and apricots, have concentrated fiber and can lead to blockages. Opt for fresh or canned varieties without added sugars instead.

Tough skins: Avoid fruits and vegetables with tough or thick skins, like apples, pears, and cucumbers, unless they are peeled or cooked thoroughly.

Gas-producing foods: Certain foods, like beans, lentils, cabbage, onions, and carbonated beverages, can produce excess gas and discomfort for some people with ileostomies.

Spicy foods: Spicy foods and strong seasonings may irritate your digestive system and cause discomfort or diarrhea.

Alcohol and caffeine: Both alcohol and caffeine can be dehydrating and may irritate your digestive tract. Limit your intake of caffeinated beverages and alcoholic drinks.

High-fat foods: While some healthy fats are okay in moderation, high-fat foods like fried foods, creamy sauces, and rich desserts can be harder to digest and may cause discomfort.

CHAPTER V: SAVORY RECIPES AND MEAL IDEAS FOR ILEOSTOMY

SAVORY RECIPES AND MEAL IDEAS FOR BREAKFAST

Classic scones with jam & clotted cream

Ingredients

350g self-raising flour, plus more for dusting

1 tsp baking powder

85g butter, cut into cubes

3 tbsp caster sugar

175ml milk

1 tsp vanilla extract

squeeze lemon juice (see tips below)

beaten egg, to glaze

jam and clotted cream, to serve

Instructions

STEP 1

Heat the oven to 220C/200C fan/gas 7. Tip the self-raising flour into a large bowl with ¼ tsp salt and the baking powder, then mix.

STEP 2

Add the butter, then rub in with your fingers until the mix looks like fine crumbs. Stir in the caster sugar.

STEP 3

Put the milk into a jug and heat in the microwave for about 30 secs until warm, but not hot. Add the vanilla extract and a squeeze of lemon juice, then set aside for a moment.

STEP 4

Put a baking tray in the oven. Make a well in the dry mix, then add the liquid and combine it quickly with a cutlery knife – it will seem pretty wet at first.

STEP 5

Scatter some flour onto the work surface and tip the dough out. Dredge the dough and your hands with a little more flour, then fold the dough over 2-3 times until it's a little smoother. Pat into a round about 4cm deep. Take a 5cm cutter (smooth-edged cutters tend to cut more cleanly, giving a better rise) and dip it into some flour. Plunge into the dough, then repeat until you have four scones. You may need to press what's left of the dough back into a round to cut out another four.

STEP 6

Brush the tops with a beaten egg, then carefully arrange on the hot baking tray. Bake for 10 mins until risen and golden on the top. Eat just warm or cold on the day of baking, generously topped with jam and clotted cream. If freezing, freeze once cool. Defrost, then put in a low oven (about 160C/140C fan/gas 3) for a few minutes to refresh.

Vegan banana bread

Ingredients

3 large black bananas

75ml vegetable oil or sunflower oil, plus extra for the tin

100g brown sugar

225g plain flour (or use self-raising flour and reduce the baking powder to 2 heaped tsp)

3 heaped tsp baking powder

3 tsp cinnamon or mixed spice

50g dried fruit or nuts (optional)

Instructions

STEP 1

Heat oven to 200C/180C fan/gas 6. Mash 3 large black peeled bananas with a fork, then mix well with 75g vegetable or sunflower oil and 100g brown sugar.

STEP 2

Add 225g plain flour, 3 heaped tsp baking powder and 3 tsp cinnamon or mixed spice, and combine well. Add 50g dried fruit or nuts, if using.

STEP 3

Bake in an oiled, lined 2lb loaf tin for 20 minutes. Check and cover with foil if the cake is browning.

STEP 4

Bake for another 20 minutes, or until a skewer comes out clean.

STEP 5

Allow to cool a little before slicing. It's delicious freshly baked, but develops a lovely gooey quality the day after.

Vegan strawberry pancakes

Ingredients

115g wholemeal spelt flour

1 tsp baking powder

1 tsp cinnamon

150ml soya milk

240g soya yogurt

1 tsp vanilla extract

drop of rapeseed oil

200g strawberries, hulled and halved or quartered if large

2 tbsp chopped pecans

a few small mint leaves, optional

Instructions

STEP 1

Mix the flour with the baking powder and cinnamon in a bowl using a balloon whisk. In a jug, whisk together the soya milk, 2 tbsp of the yogurt and vanilla extract, then whisk this into the dry Ingredients to make a thick batter.

STEP 2

Rub the oil around the pan using kitchen paper, then set the pan over a medium heat. Spoon in 1½ tbsp batter in three or four places to make small pancakes. Cook over a low heat for 1-2 mins until set, and bubbles appear on the surface, then turn the pancakes using a palette knife. Cook for another 1-2 mins until golden and cooked through. Repeat with the remaining batter to make six pancakes in total.

STEP 3

Serve three pancakes per person topped with the remaining yogurt, berries, pecans and mint leaves.

Healthy banana muffins

Ingredients

2 large eggs

150ml pot natural low-fat yogurt

50ml rapeseed oil

100g apple sauce or puréed apple

1 ripe banana, mashed

4 tbsp honey

1 tsp vanilla extract

200g wholemeal flour

50g rolled oats, plus extra for sprinkling

1 ½ tsp baking powder

1 ½ tsp bicarbonate of soda

1 ½ tsp cinnamon

100g blueberry

2 tbsp mixed seed, we used pumpkin, sunflower and flaxseed

Instructions

STEP 1

Heat oven to 180C/160C fan/gas 4. Line a 12-hole muffin tray with 12 large muffin cases. In a jug, mix the eggs, yogurt, oil, apple sauce, banana, honey and vanilla. Tip the remaining Ingredients, except the seeds, into a large bowl, add a pinch of salt and mix to combine.

STEP 2

Pour the wet Ingredients into the dry, mix briefly until you have a smooth batter, don't over mix as this will make the muffins heavy. Spoon the batter between the cases. Sprinkle the muffins with the extra oats and the seeds. Bake for 25-30 mins until golden and well risen, and a skewer inserted to the centre of a muffin comes out clean. Remove from the oven, transfer to a wire rack and leave to cool. Store in a sealed container for up to 3 days.

Breakfast casserole

Ingredients

250g chestnut mushrooms, sliced

1½ tbsp vegetable oil, plus extra for the tin (optional)

6 veggie sausages, sliced into bite-sized pieces

1 large red onion, finely sliced

2 red peppers, deseeded and sliced

8 eggs

250ml whole milk

125g cheddar, grated

10g chives, finely sliced

Instructions

STEP 1

Heat the oven to 200C/180C fan/gas 6. Fry the mushrooms in a large non-stick frying pan over a medium-high heat until the liquid has released and evaporated, about 8-10 mins. Add ½ tbsp oil and fry until golden, about 2 mins. Remove from the pan and tip into a large bowl.

STEP 2

Wipe out the pan to remove any excess liquid, then return to a medium heat. Add the remaining oil and fry the sausages until golden all over. Remove using a slotted spoon and add to the bowl with the mushrooms. Fry the onions and peppers, stirring occasionally for 8-10 mins until soft but not browned. Tip into the bowl with the sausages and mushrooms, and mix everything together to combine. Season well. Tip the sausage and veg mixture into a baking dish (around 35 x 25cm) or roasting tin. If you're using a tin, you may need to oil it to prevent the casserole from sticking.

STEP 3

Combine the eggs, milk, cheddar and chives in a large jug, season well, then pour this over the Ingredients in the dish or tin. Bake for 25-30 mins until golden and set. Leave to cool slightly before cutting into squares.

Winter breakfast hash

Ingredients

375g potatoes, cut into small chunks

1 tbsp rapeseed oil

1 onion (about 200g), chopped

½ tsp caraway seeds

2 garlic cloves, chopped

1 green pepper, deseeded and diced

200g large brussels sprouts, trimmed and sliced

2 eggs

Instructions

STEP 1

Boil the potatoes for 15 mins until tender. Meanwhile, heat the oil in a large non-stick frying pan over a medium heat and fry the onion for 8 mins, stirring frequently until it starts to colour. Add the caraway, garlic, pepper and sprouts and cook for 5 mins more with the lid on the pan so they steam at the same time.

STEP 2

Drain and lightly crush the cooked potatoes using a masher. Stir them into the vegetables and cook for 5-10 mins, turning occasionally so the mixture browns.

STEP 3

Meanwhile, poach the eggs for a few minutes for a runny yolk or until cooked to your liking. Remove from the pan using a slotted spoon. Serve each portion of hash topped with an egg.

Ackee & saltfish

Ingredients

600g boneless salted cod

2 tbsp vegetable oil

1 medium onion, finely chopped

4 garlic cloves, finely chopped

3 spring onions, thinly sliced

1 scotch bonnet pepper, deseeded and finely chopped

1 tsp dried thyme

1 tsp ground pimento (allspice)

½ red pepper, deseeded and finely chopped

½ green pepper, deseeded and finely chopped

1 large tomato, chopped

2 x 540g cans ackee, drained

Instructions

STEP 1

Put the salt cold in your pot and cover with cold water.
Bring to the boil, then boil for 5 minutes, drain and add
fresh cold water to cover.

STEP 2

Repeat this process until you're happy with the saltiness when tasted; we recommend to boil the fish three times in total for a perfect balance of salt in the fish. Drain and leave to cool. Use a fork to shred the salted cod into pieces and set aside.

STEP 3

Now you'll need a large frying pan. Pour the vegetable oil into the frying pan and place over a high heat. Once the oil is sizzling hot, turn the heat down to low-medium. Add the onion, garlic, spring onions and scotch bonnet, then cook until soft, for around 5-7 minutes.

STEP 4

Add the salted cod, dash in some black pepper, thyme and pimento, then mix it together and cook down for around 3 minutes.

STEP 5

Next, add in the red and green bell peppers, along with your tomato. Mix together and cook down for 2-3 minutes. These Ingredients help to bring a heat balance, so it's not too spicy.

STEP 6

Now you'll need to add in your ackee and dash in a little more black pepper. Fold in the ackee; the ackee is soft so it's important to fold it in very gently – nobody likes mushy ackee.

STEP 7

Once folded in, simmer for 3-5 minutes before serving.

Courgette & ricotta fritters with poached eggs & harissa yogurt

Ingredients

2 courgettes, coarsely grated

50g ricotta

1⁄2 lemon, zested

2 eggs, lightly beaten

20g parmesan or vegetarian alternative, grated

50g self-raising flour

60g Greek yogurt

1/2 tbsp rose harissa

2 tbsp olive oil

6 thin slices of pancetta (optional)

splash of white wine vinegar

2 large eggs

dill and parsley, torn, to serve 8g

Instructions

STEP 1

Line a bowl with a clean cloth and add the courgette with a pinch of salt. Set aside for 30 mins, then use the cloth to squeeze out the excess liquid. Tip the courgette into a bowl with the ricotta, lemon zest, eggs and parmesan, then stir to combine. Fold in the flour and some seasoning.

STEP 2

Stir the Greek yogurt and harissa together in a small bowl and season with a pinch of salt. Set aside.

STEP 3

Heat the oven to 180C/160C fan/gas 4. Heat the oil in a non-stick frying pan and spoon in six mounds of the courgette mixture. Cook over a medium heat for 3-4 mins each side until golden brown. Transfer to a baking sheet and bake for 10 mins.

STEP 4

Meanwhile, heat your grill to high, then cook the pancetta, if using, for 2-3 mins on each side until crisp.

STEP 5

Bring a pan of water to the boil. Drizzle a little of the vinegar into a ramekin and crack an egg into it. Swirl the water in the pan with a wooden spoon to create a whirlpool in the middle, then gently tip the egg into it and simmer for 3 mins. Repeat with the second egg. Serve three fritters stacked on each plate, topped with an egg and three slices of pancetta, alongside a dollop of the harissa yogurt, then scatter over the herbs.

Cheesy skillet hash brown & eggs

Ingredients

1 large Maris Piper potato (about 250g), coarsely grated

1 egg, beaten

1 tbsp plain flour

20g cheddar, grated

3 spring onions, finely sliced

1 tbsp vegetable oil

For the toppings

1 egg

20g cheddar, grated

1/4 tsp chilli flakes (optional)

Instructions

STEP 1

Heat the oven to 200C/180C fan/gas 6. Tip the grated potato into a clean tea towel and wring out any excess water. Transfer to a bowl and mix in the beaten egg, flour, cheese and half the spring onions. Season with plenty of salt and a grinding of black pepper.

STEP 2

Brush a 20cm ovenproof skillet or frying pan with the oil and set over a medium heat. Once hot, press the hash brown mixture into the pan using the back of a spoon, making a well in the middle. Fry for 6-8 mins until golden.

STEP 3

Transfer the hash brown to the oven and bake for 10 mins. For the toppings, break the egg into the gap and sprinkle the cheese over the hash brown. Bake for 8-10 mins until the potato is crisp and the egg white is set and the yolk runny (or cooked the way you prefer). Sprinkle over the remaining spring onions and the chilli flakes, if using.

Turmeric pancakes

Ingredients

For the pancakes

200g self raising flour

1 tsp baking powder

2 tbsp honey

¼ tsp ground ginger

½ tsp ground turmeric

200ml milk

3 eggs

25g butter, melted plus extra for frying

To serve

1-2 balls stem ginger, sliced

4 tbsp orange or lemon curd

slices of orange or mango

Instructions

STEP 1

Put all of the pancake Ingredients in a mixing bowl and whisk together until smooth and lump-free.

STEP 2

Heat a small knob of butter in a large non-stick frying pan until melted and foaming. Add 2 tbsp batter to make each pancake and swirl it round into a circle with the back of the spoon. Cook them for 2-3 mins on one side then flip them over with a spatula and cook for a further minute until golden and cooked through. Heat oven to its lowest setting, transfer the cooked pancakes to a tray and keep them warm in the oven until they've all been fried.

STEP 3

Stack the pancakes up with lemon curd, ginger and fresh fruit slices on top.

Ham & potato hash with baked beans & healthy 'fried' eggs

Ingredients

600g potato, diced

1 Cal cooking spray, for frying

2 leeks, trimmed, washed and sliced

175g lean ham, weighed after trimming and discarding any fat, chopped

2 tbsp wholegrain mustard

5 eggs

2 x 415g cans reduced sugar & salt baked beans

Instructions

STEP 1

Bring a large pan of salted water to the boil. Add the potatoes and boil for 5 mins until just tender. Drain well and leave in the colander to steam-dry.

STEP 2

Meanwhile, spray an ovenproof pan with cooking spray. Add the leeks with a splash of water and fry until very soft and squishy. Add a few more sprays of the oil, tip in the potatoes along with the ham, and fry to crisp up a little. Heat oven to 200C/180C fan/gas 6.

STEP 3

Stir in the mustard, 1 egg and a good amount of seasoning with a fork – break up some of the potatoes roughly as you do. Flatten down the mixture, spray the top with oil, and bake in the oven for 15-20 mins until the top is crisp.

STEP 4

When the hash is nearly ready, heat 200ml water in a non-stick frying pan with a lid (or use a baking sheet as a lid). When it is steaming (but before it simmers), crack in the remaining 4 eggs and cover with a lid.

Cook for 2-4 mins until the eggs are done to your liking. Meanwhile, heat the beans.

STEP 5

Lift an egg onto each plate, add a big scoop of hash and spoon on some beans.

Savoury vegan pancakes

Ingredients

150g self-raising flour

½ tsp baking powder

100g garlic & herb soft cheese alternative, (see tip below)

200ml plant milk (such as oat or soya)

½ small bunch of chives, finely chopped

1 large vine tomato, halved

4-6 portabellini or baby portobello mushrooms

1 tbsp light olive oil, plus more for cooking

a few thyme sprigs

Instructions

STEP 1

Put the flour, baking powder and a pinch of fine sea salt in a bowl and whisk briefly to combine. In a separate bowl, whisk together 50g of the garlic & herb soft cheese alternative with the milk until combined.

Stir in half the chives, then pour into the dry Ingredients, whisking to form a smooth, thick batter.

STEP 2

Heat the grill to medium high. Arrange the tomato halves, cut-side up, and the mushrooms on a tray. Season well, scatter over the thyme leaves and drizzle over 1 tbsp oil, rubbing the oil into the mushrooms. Grill for 10-15 mins until softened and the mushrooms are wilted and tender throughout.

STEP 3

Meanwhile, brush or swirl a little oil around a large non-stick frying pan and place over a medium heat. Add 2 tbsp of the batter to the pan to make small, round pancakes. Make sure they don't touch – you may need to do this in batches. Cook for 2 mins until the edges start to set and bubbles rise to the surface. Flip and cook for another 2-3 mins until light golden and cooked through. Keep the pancakes warm (underneath the tomatoes and mushrooms in the grill, or in a low oven) while you cook the remaining batter. Add a little more oil to the pan if needed. There should be 8-10 small pancakes in total.

STEP 4

Spread the remaining soft cheese alternative over the pancakes, and divide between two warmed plates. Top each with a tomato half and the mushrooms. Season and scatter over the remaining chives to serve.

No-weigh cinnamon & yogurt pancakes

Ingredients

For the dry mix

500g self raising flour

4rounded tbsp golden caster sugar

1rounded tbsp ground cinnamon

To make one batch

125g natural yogurt

1large egg

1 tbsp milk

a little butter, for frying

maple syrup or Nutella, to serve

Instructions

STEP 1

Before you go, tip the flour, sugar and cinnamon into a
bowl and mix thoroughly to distribute the cinnamon
evenly. Transfer to a rigid container and seal.

STEP 2

To make a batch of pancakes, tip the yogurt into a bowl
or jug and add the egg and milk, then mix with a fork.
Rinse the yogurt pot and dry well. Measure a scoop of
dry mix into a bowl, make a well in the centre, and add
the yogurt mixture. Beat together to make a smooth
batter.

STEP 3

Heat a frying pan with a knob of butter. Spoon
tablespoons of mixture, a little apart, into the pan and
cook until bubbles appear on the surface, about 2-3

mins. Flip them over and cook until firm to the touch, then transfer to a plate. Add a little more butter and continue to cook the pancakes until all the batter is used up. Serve with toppings of your choice.

SAVORY RECIPES AND MEAL IDEAS FOR LUNCH

Pesto chicken salad

Ingredients

50g couscous

2 tbsp pesto

2 tbsp fat-free yogurt

2 cooked skinless chicken breasts, shredded, or 200g leftover roast chicken, shredded

½ small bunch of basil, leaves picked and torn, plus a few small leaves to serve

½ cucumber, chopped

2 sundried tomatoes in oil, drained and sliced

2 Little Gem lettuces, leaves separated

2 tsp toasted pine nuts

Instructions

STEP 1

Put the couscous in a large heatproof bowl and cover with 100ml boiling water. Stir in 1 tbsp pesto. Cover and leave for 8 mins.

STEP 2

Fluff the couscous with a fork, then stir in the rest of the pesto, the yogurt and some seasoning. Toss in the chicken, basil, cucumber and tomatoes.

STEP 3

Spoon the couscous mix into the lettuce leaves and eat with your fingers, or serve over the lettuce like a salad. Scatter over the pine nuts and more basil before serving.

Easy turkey burgers

Ingredients

2 tbsp olive oil

1 large onion, finely chopped

2 garlic cloves, crushed

85g porridge oats

450g/1lb minced turkey

100g dried apricot, finely chopped

1 large carrot, grated

1 egg, beaten

cucumber slices, to serve

Instructions

STEP 1

Heat 1 tbsp oil in a pan and gently fry the onion for 5 mins until soft. Add the garlic and cook for 1 min. Add the oats and fry for 2 mins more. Tip into a bowl and set aside to cool.

STEP 2

Add the rest of the Ingredients to the cooled mixture and mix well with your hands. Season to taste and shape into 8 patties.

STEP 3

Heat oven to 200C/fan 180C/gas 6. Heat the remaining olive oil in a large, non-stick frying pan and sear the burgers on each side until well coloured (3-4 mins). Transfer to a baking sheet and cook in the oven for 10-15 mins. Serve in rolls with Tangy tomato chutney (see 'goes well with') and cucumber slices.

STEP 4

For the chutney heat 1 tbsp of olive oil in a pan and add 1 finely chopped onion. Cook for 5 mins until softened. Stir in 1 crushed garlic clove and cook for a further min. Add 1 tbsp sundried tomato paste, a 400g can good-quality chopped tomatoes and a pinch of sugar. Gently cook for 20-25 mins until rich and thick. Season to taste,

then leave to cool before serving.

Black bean & tortilla soup

Ingredients

2 tbsp olive oil

1 chopped onion

2 chopped peppers

3 crushed garlic cloves

2 tsp ground cumin

1 tsp garlic granules

1 tsp chilli powder

2 tbsp tomato purée

1l veg stock

400g can chopped tomatoes

2 tbsp cornmeal or polenta

2 tbsp chopped pickled jalapeños

2 x 400g cans black beans

jalapeño brine

4 small corn tortillas

chopped coriander, avocado, crumbled feta and pumpkin seeds, to serve, if you like

Instructions

STEP 1

Heat the olive oil in a deep pan over a medium heat. Add the onion, peppers (any colour you like) and garlic cloves with a big pinch of salt. Cook for 10 mins, until starting to soften, then add the ground cumin, garlic granules and chilli powder along with the tomato purée. Cook for 5 mins, until the purée has caramelised.

STEP 2

Pour in the veg stock, chopped tomatoes, cornmeal or polenta, chopped pickled jalapeños and black beans, along with the liquid. Add a splash of jalapeño brine and bring to a simmer. Cook for 45 mins, until thickened and reduced. Season, then scatter in the corn tortillas, cut into small strips. (Use flour tortillas if that's what you have.) Rest for 5 mins before serving. Serve with chopped coriander, avocado, crumbled feta and pumpkin seeds, if you like.

Fresh salmon niçoise

Ingredients

1 red onion (about 130g), finely chopped

2 tbsp apple cider vinegar

2 tbsp extra virgin olive oil

12 pitted Kalamata olives, quartered

2 tbsp chopped dill

2 tsp chopped tarragon leaves

400g small baby potatoes

2 eggs

320g fine green beans, trimmed

4 wild salmon fillets (about 100-125g each), defrosted
if frozen

2 x 160g Little Gem lettuces, 1 shredded

4 tomatoes, cut into wedges

Instructions

STEP 1

Combine the onion, vinegar, oil, olives and herbs in a
medium bowl.

STEP 2

Boil the potatoes in the base of a steamer for 10 mins.
Add the eggs (top up with boiling water from the kettle
if they're not submerged). Tip the green beans into a

pan and put the steamer on top, then cook for 8 mins more.

STEP 3

Remove the potatoes and eggs from the steamer, but don't drain. Add the salmon to the water and cook for 5 mins. Stir the warm potatoes into the dressing.

STEP 4

To serve, divide half the lettuce between two plates (or pile onto one platter) along with half the green beans and tomatoes, then spoon half the dressed potatoes on top. Remove and discard any skin from the salmon, then flake half the fish over the salad. Peel one egg, halve and serve one half over each salad. Chill the remaining Ingredients for the next day to eat cold. Will keep covered and chilled for up to a day.

Chicken & tzatziki wraps

Ingredients

1 cucumber, three-quarters deseeded and coarsely grated, the rest halved and sliced

250g Greek yogurt

500g chicken breast, thinly sliced

2tbsp olive oil

4 wholemeal wraps

4 large ripe tomatoes, thinly sliced

Instructions

STEP 1

For the tzatziki, tip the grated cucumber and yogurt into a bowl, mix well and season. Set aside. Season the chicken with salt and pepper and rub with 1 tbsp of the olive oil. Heat the remaining oil in a pan over a medium heat. Cook the chicken for 8-10 mins until cooked through and golden brown.

STEP 2

Warm the wraps in a dry pan or microwave. Spread 2 tbsp of the tzatziki onto each wrap, top with the chicken, tomatoes and sliced cucumber. Season with a little more pepper, if you like, then fold the sides of the wrap over the filling, roll up tightly and serve.

Wild salmon veggie bowl

Ingredients

2 carrots

1large courgette

2 cooked beetroot, diced

2 tbsp balsamic vinegar

⅓ small pack dill, chopped, plus some extra fronts (optional)

1small red onion, finely chopped

280g poached or canned wild salmon

2 tbsp capers in vinegar, rinsed

Instructions

STEP 1

Shred the carrots and courgette into long spaghetti strips with a julienne peeler or spiralizer, and pile onto two plates.

STEP 2

Stir the beetroot, balsamic vinegar, chopped dill and red onion together in a small bowl, then spoon on top of the veg. Flake over chunks of the salmon and scatter with the capers and extra dill, if you like.

Summer carrot, tarragon & white bean soup

Ingredients

1 tbsp rapeseed oil

2 large leeks, well washed, halved lengthways and finely sliced

700g carrots, chopped

1.4l hot reduced-salt vegetable bouillon (we used Marigold)

4 garlic cloves, finely grated

2 x 400g cans cannellini beans in water

⅔ small pack tarragon, leaves roughly chopped

Instructions

STEP 1

Heat the oil over a medium heat in a large pan and fry the leeks and carrots for 5 mins to soften.

STEP 2

Pour over the stock, stir in the garlic, the beans with their liquid, and three-quarters of the tarragon, then cover and simmer for 15 mins or until the veg is just tender. Stir in the remaining tarragon before serving.

Ricotta, broccoli, & new potato frittata

Ingredients

100g new potatoes

200g long-stem broccoli

200g green beans, trimmed and halved

400g can mixed beans, drained

3 tsp rapeseed oil

2 garlic cloves, crushed

pinch of chilli flakes, cumin seeds or fennel seeds

4 large eggs

50g ricotta

1 tsp sherry vinegar

½ small bunch of basil, roughly chopped (optional)

Instructions

STEP 1

Boil the potatoes for 10-15 mins until tender. Add the broccoli for the last 2 mins of cooking. Drain and thickly slice the potatoes.

STEP 2

Meanwhile, put the green beans and mixed beans in a pan and cover with water. Bring to a simmer and cook for 3-4 mins, or until the green beans are tender. Drain and leave to steam-dry in the pan.

STEP 3

Heat the grill to high. Heat 2 tsp of the oil in a medium non-stick frying pan and fry the garlic for 1 min, then add the chilli flakes or cumin or fennel seeds and cook for 1 min more. Add the potatoes, broccoli and seasoning, and toss to coat in the flavoured oil.

STEP 4

Beat the eggs in a jug, season and pour over the potato mix. Cook over a medium heat for 2 mins, or until the base is set. Dollop teaspoons of the ricotta on top, then grill for 4-5 mins until cooked through.

STEP 5

Meanwhile, drizzle another 1 tsp oil over the bean mixture with the vinegar. Stir in the basil, if using, and season. Slice the frittata into four wedges, and serve two with half the bean salad on the side. Chill the remaining wedges and bean salad to use in the lunchboxes below.

Kale soup

Ingredients

2 tbsp rapeseed oil

3 onions (320g), finely chopped

3 garlic cloves, finely grated

125g celery, chopped

2 yellow peppers, deseeded and diced

2 tsp smoked paprika

400g can chopped tomatoes

2 tsp dried oregano

1 litre hot vegetable stock, made with 3 tsp bouillon powder

150g wholemeal penne

200g green beans, trimmed and cut into short lengths

200g cavolo nero (kale), thinly sliced

160g cherry tomatoes

30g pack of basil, chopped

80g vegetarian Italian-style hard cheese, finely grated

Instructions

STEP 1

Heat the oil in a large pan over a medium heat and fry the onions and garlic for 5 mins, then add the celery and peppers. Fry for another 5 mins, adding the smoked paprika in the last minute. Stir in the tomatoes, oregano and stock. Bring to the boil.

STEP 2

Tip in the penne, green beans and kale, bring back to the boil and cook over a medium heat for 10 mins. Stir in the cherry tomatoes and basil, and cook for a few minutes more until the tomatoes have burst.

STEP 3

To serve, spoon two portions of the soup into shallow bowls and sprinkle over half the cheese. Keep the remainder for another day. Will keep chilled in an airtight container for up to four days or frozen for up to three months. Reheat in a pan over a low-medium heat until piping hot, then serve with the remaining cheese.

Beetroot, cumin & coriander soup with yogurt and hazelnut dukkah

Ingredients

2 tbsp olive oil

2 red onions, cut into wedges

1kg raw beetroot, peeled and cut into wedges

1 tsp chilli flakes

1 tbsp cumin seeds, plus 1 tsp

1 ½ tbsp coriander seeds

1 tbsp red wine vinegar

1.2l vegetable stock (we used Bouillon)

30g hazelnuts

1 tbsp sesame seeds

4 tbsp natural yogurt

Instructions

STEP 1

Heat the oil in a large saucepan. Add the onions, beetroot and a pinch of salt and cook for 10 mins, then turn up the heat and add the chilli flakes and 1 tbsp each of the cumin and coriander seeds. Cook until aromatic, then add the vinegar and give everything a good stir. Pour in the stock and bring to the boil, then cover and simmer for 45 mins-1 hr until a knife can be easily inserted into a beetroot wedge; uncover the pan halfway through cooking to reduce the soup.

STEP 2

Meanwhile, make the dukkah. Put the hazelnuts, sesame seeds and the remaining cumin and coriander into a dry frying pan and gently toast until the hazelnuts are golden. Add a pinch of salt and crush with a pestle and mortar (alternatively, use a knife to roughly chop the nuts).

STEP 3

Blitz the soup with a hand blender and season to taste. Divide between four bowls, then top with a swirl of the yogurt and a sprinkling of hazelnut dukkah.

Chicken satay salad

Ingredients

1 tbsp tamari

1 tsp medium curry powder

¼ tsp ground cumin

1 garlic clove, finely grated

1 tsp clear honey

2 skinless chicken breast fillets (or use turkey breast)

1 tbsp crunchy peanut butter (choose a sugar-free version with no palm oil, if possible)

1 tbsp sweet chilli sauce

1 tbsp lime juice

sunflower oil, for wiping the pan

2 Little Gem lettuce hearts, cut into wedges

¼ cucumber, halved and sliced

1 banana shallot, halved and thinly sliced

coriander, chopped

seeds from ½ pomegranate

Instructions

STEP 1

Pour the tamari into a large dish and stir in the curry
powder, cumin, garlic and honey. Mix well. Slice the
chicken breasts in half horizontally to make 4 fillets in

total, then add to the marinade and mix well to coat. Set aside in the fridge for at least 1 hr, or overnight, to allow the flavours to penetrate the chicken.

STEP 2

Meanwhile, mix the peanut butter with the chilli sauce, lime juice, and 1 tbsp water to make a spoonable sauce. When ready to cook the chicken, wipe a large non-stick frying pan with a little oil. Add the chicken and cook, covered with a lid, for 5-6 mins on a medium heat, turning the fillets over for the last min, until cooked but still moist. Set aside, covered, to rest for a few mins.

STEP 3

While the chicken rests, toss the lettuce wedges with the cucumber, shallot, coriander and pomegranate, and pile onto plates. Spoon over a little sauce. Slice the chicken, pile on top of the salad and spoon over the remaining sauce. Eat while the chicken is still warm.

The best spaghetti bolognese recipe

Ingredients

1 tbsp olive oil

4 rashers smoked streaky bacon, finely chopped

2 medium onions, finely chopped

2 carrots, trimmed and finely chopped

2 celery sticks, finely chopped

2 garlic cloves finely chopped

2-3 sprigs rosemary leaves picked and finely chopped

500g beef mince

For the bolognese sauce

2 x 400g tins plum tomatoes

small pack basil leaves picked, ¾ finely chopped and the rest left whole for garnish

1 tsp dried oregano

2 fresh bay leaves

2 tbsp tomato purée

1 beef stock cube

1 red chilli deseeded and finely chopped (optional)

125ml red wine

6 cherry tomatoes sliced in half

To season and serve

75g parmesan grated, plus extra to serve

400g spaghetti

crusty bread to serve (optional)

Instructions

STEP 1

Put a large saucepan on a medium heat and add 1 tbsp olive oil.

STEP 2

Add 4 finely chopped bacon rashers and fry for 10 mins until golden and crisp.

STEP 3

Reduce the heat and add the 2 onions, 2 carrots, 2 celery sticks, 2 garlic cloves and the leaves from 2-3 sprigs rosemary, all finely chopped, then fry for 10 mins. Stir the veg often until it softens.

STEP 4

Increase the heat to medium-high, add 500g beef mince and cook stirring for 3-4 mins until the meat is browned all over.

STEP 5

Add 2 tins plum tomatoes, the finely chopped leaves from ¾ small pack basil, 1 tsp dried oregano, 2 bay leaves, 2 tbsp tomato purée, 1 beef stock cube, 1 deseeded and finely chopped red chilli (if using), 125ml red wine and 6 halved cherry tomatoes. Stir with a wooden spoon, breaking up the plum tomatoes.

STEP 6

Bring to the boil, reduce to a gentle simmer and cover with a lid. Cook for 1 hr 15 mins stirring occasionally, until you have a rich, thick sauce.

STEP 7

Add the 75g grated parmesan, check the seasoning and stir.

STEP 8

When the bolognese is nearly finished, cook 400g spaghetti following the pack instructions.

STEP 9

Drain the spaghetti and either stir into the bolognese sauce, or serve the sauce on top. Serve with more grated parmesan, the remaining basil leaves and crusty bread, if you like.

Spicy chicken & avocado wraps

Ingredients

1 chicken breast (approx 180g), thinly sliced at an angle

generous squeeze juice 0.5 lime

½ tsp mild chilli powder

1 garlic clove, chopped

1 tsp olive oil

2 seeded wraps

1 avocado, halved and stoned

1 roasted red pepper from a jar, sliced

a few sprigs coriander, chopped

Instructions

STEP 1

Mix the chicken with the lime juice, chilli powder and garlic.

STEP 2

Heat the oil in a non-stick frying pan then fry the chicken for a couple of mins – it will cook very quickly so keep an eye on it. Meanwhile, warm the wraps following the pack instructions or, if you have a gas hob, heat them over the flame to slightly char them. Do not let them dry out or they are difficult to roll.

STEP 3

Squash half an avocado onto each wrap, add the peppers to the pan to warm them through then pile onto the wraps with the chicken, and sprinkle over the coriander. Roll up, cut in half and eat with your fingers.

Carrot & lentil soup with feta

Ingredients

2 tbsp rapeseed oil

3 onions, chopped (420g)

5 garlic cloves, chopped

750g carrots, sliced

1 tbsp smoked paprika

1 tbsp ground coriander

1 tbsp thyme leaves

300g red lentils

1.3l boiling vegetable stock, made with 2 tsp bouillon powder

2 x 400g cans chickpeas

150g feta, crumbled

Instructions

STEP 1

Heat the oil in a large pan over a medium heat and fry the onions for 10 mins, stirring frequently until starting to turn golden. Add the garlic and carrots, and cook a few minutes more, then stir in the spices, thyme and lentils.

STEP 2

Pour in the stock, then cover and simmer for 20 mins until the lentils are pulpy and tender. Remove from the heat and roughly blitz using a hand blender – you don't want it to be completely smooth. Stir in the chickpeas and the liquid from the cans, and reheat the soup. Serve two bowls straightaway, each topped with 25g of the crumbled feta. Leave the remaining soup to cool before keeping chilled for up to four days. Reheat in a pan over a low heat until piping hot, then scatter over 25g of the remaining feta for each portion.

SAVORY RECIPES AND MEAL IDEAS FOR DINNER

Cardamom chicken with lime leaves

Ingredients

For the curry

2 tbsp rapeseed oil

1 large onion, finely chopped

4 large garlic cloves, grated

2 tbsp finely grated fresh ginger

12 cardamom pods, seeds removed and lightly crushed

4 cloves

1 cinnamon stick

2 tsp turmeric

½-1 tsp ground white pepper

1 tsp ground coriander

1 tsp ground cumin

1 red chilli halved, deseeded and finely sliced

400g can chopped tomatoes

1 tbsp mango chutney

2 tsp vegetable bouillon powder

1 aubergine, cubed

12 skinless boneless chicken thighs (about 1kg)

4 small fresh or dried lime leaves

1 green pepper, halved, deseeded and sliced

For the spiced rice & lentils

125g brown basmati rice

100g dried red lentils

1 tsp cumin seeds

1 tsp turmeric

1 tsp vegetable bouillon powder

Instructions

STEP 1

Heat the oil in a large, wide pan, add the onion and fry for 5 mins until softened, stirring every now and then. Stir in the garlic, ginger, cardamom, cloves and cinnamon, and cook for 5 mins more, stirring frequently. Add all the remaining spices with the chilli, stir briefly over the heat then add the tomatoes with 1 can of water, the chutney and bouillon.

STEP 2

Stir in the aubergine, bring to the boil then cover the pan and simmer for 15 mins. Stir well, and add the chicken and lime leaves. Push them under the liquid and scatter over the green pepper. Cover the pan and leave to cook for 40 mins. Remove the chicken, shred in to medium-sized pieces and return to the sauce.

STEP 3

Meanwhile, make the rice. Put all the Ingredients in a medium pan with 750ml water. Bring to the boil, then cover and cook for 20 mins. Turn off the heat and leave for 5 mins to absorb any excess moisture. Serve with the curry.

One-pot chicken & chickpea pilau

Ingredients

1 tbsp olive oil

4 chicken thighs, skin removed and trimmed of fat

2 large leeks, thinly sliced

2 garlic cloves, crushed

400g can chickpeas in water, drained and rinsed

grated zest of 1 lemon

200g easy-cook brown rice

450ml chicken stock

1 head broccoli, broken into florets

Instructions

STEP 1

Heat a large, lidded frying pan or flameproof casserole and add the oil. Fry the chicken thighs for 2 mins, turning halfway through cooking, until lightly coloured, then lift onto a plate. Add the leeks to the pan and stir-fry for 3 mins, then add the garlic and tip in the chickpeas, most of the lemon zest and rice. Stir together until well mixed.

STEP 2

Nestle the chicken in the rice mix. Pour over the stock and season lightly. Cover and cook on a low heat for 20 mins until the chicken is nearly cooked through and the rice has absorbed nearly all the liquid. Sit the broccoli on top of the rice, cover and continue to cook until the rice and broccoli are tender and the chicken cooked. Sprinkle with the remaining lemon zest to serve.

Creamy chicken, squash & pecan pasta

Ingredients

1l chicken stock

½ butternut squash, peeled and chopped into small chunks

2 chicken breasts

400g pasta (we used casarecce)

50g cream cheese

75g pecans, chopped

small pack flat-leaf parsley, chopped

25g parmesan grated, plus extra to serve

Instructions

STEP 1

Pour the stock into a pan and bring to a simmer. Add the squash and chicken, cover and bubble gently for 15 mins, or until the chicken and squash are cooked. If the chicken cooks first, remove from the pan, set aside and keep boiling the squash until tender. Scoop the squash out with a slotted spoon, leaving just the stock in the pan.

STEP 2

Bring the stock back to the boil and add the pasta; the liquid should just cover the pasta. Cook, stirring regularly, until the pasta is just tender and most of the stock has been absorbed (top up with water if necessary). Shred the chicken.

STEP 3

Return the squash to the pan and add the cream cheese, pecans, parsley and parmesan. Simmer for another min or two, then add the chicken. Season and serve with extra parmesan, if you like.

Pulled chicken salad

Ingredients

1 small roasted chicken, about 1kg

½ red cabbage, cored and finely sliced

3 carrots, coarsley grated or finely shredded

5 spring onions, finely sliced on the diagonal

2 red chillies, halved and thinly sliced

small bunch coriander, roughly chopped, including stalks

2 heaped tbsp roasted salted peanuts, roughly crushed

For the dressing

3 ½ tbsp hoisin sauce

1 ½ tbsp toasted sesame oil

Instructions

STEP 1

Combine the dressing Ingredients in a small bowl and set aside.

STEP 2

Remove all the meat from the chicken, shred into large chunks and pop in a large bowl. Add the cabbage, carrots, spring onions, chillies and half the coriander. Toss together with the dressing and pile onto a serving plate, then scatter over the remaining coriander and peanuts.

Cod & olive tagine with brown rice

Ingredients

3 tbsp rapeseed oil

2 red onions (about 320g), chopped

250g swede, finely chopped

2 carrots (about 200g), finely chopped

3 strips of lemon peel, finely chopped

4 garlic cloves, thinly sliced

1 tsp ground cinnamon

1 tsp cumin seeds

2 tsp ground coriander

400g can chopped tomatoes

2 tbsp tomato purée

300ml vegetable stock, made with 1½ tsp bouillon powder

12 pitted green olives, halved lengthways

250g easy-cook brown rice

4 frozen skinless cod fillets (about 360g)

⅓ pack of coriander, chopped

Instructions

STEP 1

Heat the oil in a large pan over a medium heat and fry the onions, swede, carrots, lemon peel and garlic for 10 mins, stirring frequently. Add the spices and stir briefly.

STEP 2

Stir in the tomatoes, tomato purée, stock and olives. Cover and cook for 25 mins.

STEP 3

Boil the rice following pack instructions. Stir the tomato mixture well, then nestle in the frozen cod fillets. Cover and cook for 20 mins until the fish is cooked through. Scatter with the coriander. Serve half with half the cooked rice. Leave the rest of the tagine and rice to cool, then keep chilled for up to three days. Reheat the tagine in a pan over a low heat until piping hot, and reheat the rice in the microwave until completely heated through.

Olive, cauliflower & harissa pasta

Ingredients

1 tbsp olive oil

1 small cauliflower, broken into small florets, stalks and leaves finely chopped

1 tbsp tomato purée

200g cherry tomatoes, halved

2 garlic cloves, crushed

25g pitted green olives, halved

2 tbsp rose harissa

150g dairy-free wholemeal pasta of your choice (such as pappardelle; gluten-free if needed)

small handful of parsley, finely chopped

Instructions

STEP 1

Heat the oil in a large frying pan over a medium-high heat and tip in the cauliflower florets, stalks and leaves. Season, cover and fry for 8-10 mins, shaking the pan now and then, until lightly browned and softened. Stir the tomato purée and tomatoes, cover and cook for 5 mins more until the tomatoes have burst. Add the garlic, olives and harissa, and cook for 2-3 mins until fragrant.

STEP 2

Meanwhile, cook the pasta following pack instructions. Drain, reserving a mugful of the water. Stir the pasta and a splash of the water into the tomato mixture. Season, scatter over the parsley and serve.

Lemon & spinach rice with feta

Ingredients

1 tbsp rapeseed oil

2 onions (320g), finely chopped

3 large garlic cloves, sliced

300g easy-cook brown rice

700ml hot vegetable stock, made with 1 tsp bouillon powder

400g frozen spinach

15g dill, finely chopped

1 lemon, zested, 1/2 juiced, 1/2 cut into 4 wedges

40g walnuts, chopped

75g feta, crumbled

Instructions

STEP 1

Heat the oil in a large pan over a medium heat and fry the onions and garlic for 10 mins, stirring often until softened.

STEP 2

Tip in the rice, then the stock, frozen spinach and half each of the dill and lemon zest. Cover, reduce the heat to low and cook for 25 mins until the rice is tender.

STEP 3

Scatter over the remaining dill and lemon zest, the nuts and feta, then gently toss together along with the lemon juice. Serve half of the rice straightaway with two lemon wedges on the side for squeezing over. Leave the rest of the rice to cool completely and keep chilled for up to three days. Reheat in the microwave until piping hot, then serve with the remaining lemon wedges.

Salmon with leeks & parsnip mash

Ingredients

x salmon fillets

juice and finely grated zest 1 lemon

2 tbsp thyme leaves

1kg parsnips, chopped

4 tbsp fromage frais

1 tbsp olive oil

2 leeks, thinly sliced

Instructions

STEP 1

Heat oven to 200C/180C fan/gas 6. Place the salmon pieces into a roasting tin, squeeze over the lemon juice and scatter with ½ the zest. Season and sprinkle over ½ the thyme. Roast for 15 mins until salmon is cooked through.

STEP 2

Meanwhile, bring a lightly salted pan of water to the boil and cook the parsnips for 15 mins, until tender. Drain well, then mash with the remaining lemon zest and the fromage frais. Keep warm.

STEP 3

Heat the oil in a non-stick frying pan. Cook the leeks over a medium heat for 6-8 mins, adding a splash of water and covering with a lid after 5 mins, until soft. Stir the leeks into the mash and serve with the salmon, scattered with the remaining thyme leaves.

Roast cauliflower & hazelnut pilaf

Ingredients

2 tbsp olive oil

1 onion, chopped

2 garlic cloves, crushed

5cm piece ginger, grated

2 tbsp garam masala

300g brown basmati rice

700ml hot vegetable stock

3 curry leaves

250g cauliflower, broken into florets

2 tbsp medium curry powder

handful coriander, chopped

100g toasted hazelnut, chopped

150ml pot natural yogurt, to serve

Instructions

STEP 1

Heat oven to 200C/180C fan/gas 6. Heat 1 tbsp of the oil in a large pan, add the onion and cook for 5 mins until golden. Add the garlic, ginger, garam masala and rice, and cook for a few more mins. Add the stock and curry leaves, and season. Bring to the boil, then reduce heat to low. Cover and simmer for 40 mins.

STEP 2

Toss the cauliflower in the curry powder and remaining oil, season and put on a baking sheet. Roast in the oven for 40 mins until tender.

STEP 3

Remove the rice pan from the heat and leave for 5 mins, then gently stir through the roasted cauliflower, coriander and toasted hazelnuts. Serve with natural yogurt.

Roasted chickpea wraps

Ingredients

2 x 400g cans chickpeas

2 tsp olive oil

2 tsp ground cumin

2 tsp smoked paprika

2 avocados, stoned, peeled and chopped

juice 1 lime

small pack coriander, chopped

8 soft corn tortillas

1 small iceberg lettuce, shredded

150g pot natural yogurt

480g jar roasted red peppers, chopped

Instructions

STEP 1

Heat oven to 220C/200C fan/gas 7. Drain the chickpeas and put in a large bowl. Add the olive oil, cumin and paprika. Stir the chickpeas well to coat, then spread them onto a large baking tray and roast for 20-25 mins or until starting to crisp – give the tray a shake halfway through cooking to ensure they roast evenly. Remove from the oven and season to taste.

STEP 2

Toss the chopped avocados with the lime juice and chopped coriander, then set aside until serving. Warm the tortillas following pack instructions, then pile in the avocado, lettuce, yogurt, peppers and toasted chickpeas at the table.

Roasted root & chickpea salad

Ingredients

4 carrots, peeled and cut into rough chunks

1 celeriac, peeled and cut into rough chunks

1 butternut squash, peeled and cut into rough chunks

1 tbsp smoked paprika

1 tbsp ground cumin

1 tsp cinnamon

1 tsp turmeric

4 tbsp olive oil

4 raw beetroot, peeled and cut into rough chunks

2 x 400g cans chickpeas, drained and rinsed

1 small red onion, thinly sliced

2 tbsp red wine vinegar (check the label if you're vegan)

pinch of sugar

1 small pack coriander, roughly chopped

1 small pack mint, roughly chopped

50g almonds, toasted and roughly chopped

Instructions

STEP 1

Heat oven to 220C/200C fan/gas 7. Put the carrots, celeriac and squash in a large bowl. Sprinkle over ¾ of the spices and ¾ of the oil. Toss to combine and season. Transfer to two large roasting trays. Add the beetroot to the same bowl, and toss in the remaining oil, spices and some seasoning, then divide between the roasting trays (coating the beetroot separately will stop everything turning purple). Roast the veg for 45 mins or until tender, tossing halfway. Add the chickpeas to the tray, stir, then return to the oven for 5 mins.

STEP 2

Meanwhile, mix the onion with the vinegar, sugar and some seasoning. Set aside to pickle.

STEP 3

Transfer the roasted vegetables to a sharing platter, stir through the pickled onions and their vinegar, the herbs and almonds, and serve.

Sweet potato & chestnut roast with tangy tomato sauce

Ingredients

For the loaf

1 tbsp rapeseed oil, plus a dash for greasing

2 onions, finely chopped

1 large sweet potato, about 325g, coarsely grated

3 garlic cloves, crushed

180g pack cooked chestnuts

2 tbsp fresh thyme leaves, plus extra for sprinkling

1 tbsp tamari

1 large egg

For the sauce

2 tsp wholemeal flour

300ml vegetable bouillon made with 1 tsp powder

2 tbsp tomato purée

1 tbsp apple cider vinegar

pinch mild chilli powder

Instructions

STEP 1

Heat oven to 180C/160C fan/gas 4. Grease and line the base and sides of a 1lb (500g) loaf tin with baking parchment. Heat the oil in a large non-stick sauté pan and fry the onions for 10 mins until golden, stirring every now and then. Add the grated potato and garlic and cook for 5 mins more until the potatoes have softened.

STEP 2

Tip into a bowl, (reserve the pan) and add two-thirds of the chestnuts crushing them up as you go, then stir in the thyme, tamari and egg. Press into the loaf tin, roughly break the remaining nuts and arrange them on top then bake for 45 mins.

STEP 3

For the sauce mix the flour with a little of the bouillon to make a very wet paste. Return the pan to the heat and add all the Ingredients, including the flour mix and stir over a high heat until well mixed and thickened. Keep simmering for a good 10 mins then taste as it should now be tangy rather than vinegary. If it is too sharp return to the heat and boil a little longer.

STEP 4

Carefully take the loaf from the tin and remove the paper. Scatter with thyme.

Cauliflower & squash fritters with mint & feta dip

Ingredients

100g gram (chickpea) flour

1 tsp turmeric

1 tsp ground cumin

small bunch coriander, finely chopped (optional)

oil, for shallow frying

150g natural yogurt

1 garlic clove, crushed

75g vegetarian feta, mashed

2 tbsp finely chopped mint

pitta breads and salad, to serve

For the roast cauliflower & squash base

1 cauliflower, split into florets, the stalk cut into cubes

½ large butternut squash, cut into cubes

1 tbsp oil

Instructions

STEP 1

Heat oven to 180C/160C fan/gas 4. Toss the cauliflower and squash in oil and spread it out on a large oven tray. Roast for 25 mins, or until tender. If you're making the base ahead of time, you can leave it to cool at this stage then freeze in an airtight container for up to a month. (Defrost fully before using in the next step.)

STEP 2

Put the flour in a bowl and gradually stir in 125-150ml water to make a batter as thick as double cream. Stir in the turmeric and cumin and some seasoning. Break up the cauliflower and squash a little and mix it gently into the batter. Add the coriander, if using.

STEP 3

Heat a little oil in a frying pan and when it is hot, drop 2 heaped tbsps of the mixture into the pan, spaced apart. Fry until the fritters are dark golden, about 2-3 mins each side. Remove, keep warm and repeat with the remaining batter.

STEP 4

Mix the yogurt with the garlic, feta and mint. Serve the fritters with the mint & feta dip, some salad and pitta breads.

SAVORY RECIPES AND MEAL IDEAS FOR SNACK

Cheese & rosemary biscuits

Ingredients

80g wholemeal flour

80g plain flour

100g cold butter, chopped

100g cheddar, finely grated

1 small rosemary sprig, leaves finely chopped

1 large egg yolk

Instructions

STEP 1

Heat oven to 180C/160C fan/ gas 4. Put the flours in a bowl and rub in the butter until it resembles breadcrumbs. Stir in the cheese and rosemary, then add the yolk and mix in using a fork. When the mix starts to clump together, use your hands to knead to a smooth dough.

STEP 2

Take walnut-sized pieces of dough, roll into balls and place on one or two lined baking trays. Flatten slightly with a fork, then bake for 12-14 mins. Alternatively, roll out between sheets of baking parchment and cut into shapes, then bake as before. Cool on the baking sheet for a few mins before moving to a wire rack to

cool completely. Store in an airtight container for up to
a week.

Rhubarb & date chutney

Ingredients

50g fresh root ginger, grated

300ml red wine vinegar

500g eating apple, peeled and finely chopped

200g pitted date, chopped

200g dried cranberries or raisins

1 tbsp mustard seed

1 tbsp curry powder

400g light muscovado sugar

700g rhubarb, sliced into 2cm chunks

500g red onion

Instructions

STEP 1

Put the onions in a large pan with the ginger and vinegar. Bring to the boil, then simmer for 10 mins. Add the rest of the Ingredients, except the rhubarb, plus 2 tsp salt to the pan and bring to the boil, stirring. Simmer, uncovered, for about 10 mins until the apples are tender.

STEP 2

Stir in the rhubarb and cook, uncovered, until the chutney is thick and jammy, about 15-20 mins. Leave the chutney to sit for about 10-15 mins, then spoon into warm, clean jars, and seal. Label the jars when cool. Keep for at least a month before eating.

Sesame prawn toast

Ingredients

200g prawns, peeled and cleaned

1 garlic clove, roughly chopped

1 tsp finely grated ginger

1 egg white

½ tsp golden caster sugar

1 tsp light soy sauce, plus extra to serve

2 spring onions, very finely chopped

3 slices white bread, crusts removed

sesame oil, for brushing

1 egg, lightly beaten

100g sesame seeds

groundnut or sunflower oil, for shallow frying

Instructions

STEP 1

Put the prawns, garlic, ginger, egg white, sugar and soy in a food processor and blitz to a paste. Stir in the spring onion. Scrape into a bowl, cover and chill for 30 mins.

STEP 2

Brush one side of each piece of bread with sesame oil. Spread the prawn mixture on top, taking it right to the edges of the bread. Brush the beaten egg carefully over the top and sides and sprinkle liberally with sesame seeds so they stick all over.

STEP 3

Heat 2-3cm oil in a sauté pan or deep frying pan until hot, and cook each piece of bread (it's easier to cook one at a time), unspread-side down for 1½ mins, then carefully turn over and cook for 1-2 mins on the prawn side or until the sesame seeds are golden and the prawn paste cooked through. Cut each piece into four triangles. Serve with soy sauce (or a sweet & sour sauce) for dipping, if you like.

Halloumi fries

Ingredients

170g pot Greek yogurt

1 lemon, zested, then cut into wedges for squeezing

1 tbsp rose harissa

3 tbsp za'atar, plus extra for sprinkling

75g plain flour

2 x 250g blocks halloumi, cut into fries

oil, for frying

handful mint, leaves torn

Instructions

STEP 1

Mix the yogurt with the lemon zest and some seasoning, then swirl through the harissa so that you have pockets of hot and cool in the dip.

STEP 2

On a plate, stir the za'atar into the flour, then roll the halloumi in the mixture so that it's evenly coated. Heat the oil in a shallow, heavy-bottomed pan or casserole dish until 180C on a cooking thermometer, or a piece of bread browns in 20 secs. Working in batches, carefully lower the halloumi into the oil and cook for 2 mins until crisp and golden, then drain on kitchen paper.

STEP 3

Sprinkle over the mint and za'atar, and serve with the lemon wedges and the spicy yogurt for dipping.

Cauliflower cheese cakes

Ingredients

oil, for greasing

½ head of cauliflower, cut into florets (about 200g)

1 slice brown bread, ripped into chunks

1 egg

50g grated cheddar

a few chives, snipped

Instructions

STEP 1

Heat the oven to 180C/160 fan/gas 4 and line a baking tray with foil. Brush with a little oil. Put the cauliflower in a steamer over boiling water and cook for around 8 mins or until tender. Allow to cool.

STEP 2

Put the bread into a food processor and blitz to crumbs. Add the cauliflower, egg, grated cheese, chives and a little black pepper and pulse until you have a chunky consistency.

STEP 3

Form into 8 patties. Arrange them on the baking tray and cook for 20 mins until golden and starting to crisp around the edges.

Spicy chicken nuggets

Ingredients

500g chicken thighs

150ml natural yogurt

3 tbsp tikka masala curry paste

100g breadcrumbs

50g crispy onions

spray oil

100g mayonnaise

1 lime, zested and cut into wedges to serve

2 tbsp mango chutney

Instructions

STEP 1

Cut the chicken thighs into nugget sized pieces then put in a bowl with the yogurt and curry paste. Cover and leave in the fridge to marinate for 2 hrs.

STEP 2

Heat the oven to 200C/180C fan/gas 6. In a baking dish mix together the breadcrumbs and dried onions. Turn the marinated chicken pieces in the breadcrumb mix

then put on a baking tray and spray each nugget with
the oil (this will help them to get crispy). Roast for 25
mins.

STEP 3

Meanwhile mix the mayonnaise with the lime zest and swirl in the mango chutney. Serve the nuggets with the mayo and lime wedges for squeezing.

Honeycomb

Ingredients

butter, for the tin

200g caster sugar

5 tbsp golden syrup

2 tsp bicarbonate of soda

Instructions

STEP 1

Butter a 20cm square tin. Stir the caster sugar and golden syrup together in a deep saucepan over a gentle heat until the sugar has melted. Try not to let the mixture bubble until the sugar grains have disappeared.

STEP 2

Once completely melted, turn up the heat a little and simmer until you have an amber coloured caramel (this won't take long), then as quickly as you can, turn off the heat, tip in the bicarbonate of soda and beat in with a wooden spoon until it has all disappeared and the mixture is foaming. Scrape into the tin immediately – be careful, the mixture will be very hot.

STEP 3

The mixture will continue bubbling in the tin, simply leave it and in about 1 hr-1 hr 30 mins the honeycomb will be hard and ready to crumble or snap into chunks.

Egg & rocket pizzas

Ingredients

2 seeded wraps

a little olive oil, for brushing

1 roasted red pepper, from a jar

2 tomatoes

2 tbsp tomato purée

1 tbsp chopped dill

2 tbsp chopped parsley

2 eggs

65g pack rocket

½ red onion, very thinly sliced

Instructions

STEP 1

Heat oven to 200C/180C fan/gas 6. Lay the tortillas on two baking sheets, brush sparingly with the oil then bake for 3 mins. Meanwhile chop the pepper and tomatoes and mix with the tomato purée, seasoning and herbs. Turn the tortillas over and spread with the tomato mixture, leaving the centre free from any large

pieces of pepper or tomato.

STEP 2

Break an egg into the centre then return to the oven for 10 mins or until the egg is just set and the tortilla is crispy round the edges. Serve scattered with the rocket and onion.

Pistachio & cranberry cookies

Ingredients

175g butter, softened

85g golden caster sugar

½ tsp vanilla extract

225g plain flour

75g pistachios

75g dried cranberries

Instructions

STEP 1

Mix the butter, sugar and vanilla extract with a wooden spoon. stir in the flour, then tip in the pistachios and cranberries – you might need to get your hands in at this stage to bring the mix together as a dough. Halve the dough and shape each half into a log about 5cm across. Wrap in cling film, then chill for 1 hr or freeze for up to 3 months.

STEP 2

Heat oven to 180C/160C fan/gas 4. slice the logs into 1cm-thick rounds, place on a baking tray lined with baking parchment and bake for 12-15 mins. Cool completely on the tray.

Manchego & chorizo melting biscuits

Ingredients

125g plain flour

½ tsp sweet smoked paprika

1 tsp fennel seeds, crushed

100g cold salted butter, cubed

100g manchego, grated

80g chorizo, very finely chopped

Instructions

STEP 1

Put the flour, paprika and fennel seeds in a food processor and blitz with the butter until it resembles fine breadcrumbs. Add the manchego and chopped chorizo and blitz again until a dough forms. Roll into a 4cm log and wrap in baking parchment. Chill in the freezer for 30-40 mins until firm.

STEP 2

Heat the oven to 180C/160C fan/gas 4. Unwrap the dough and slice into 5mm-thick biscuits. Lay on a lined baking sheet well spaced apart (they will spread in the oven). Bake for 15-20 mins until golden. Leave to cool. Will keep in an airtight container for three days.

Smoky chorizo sausage rolls

Ingredients

320g ready-rolled all-butter puff pastry

6 chorizo-style sausages (400g)

1 medium egg, beaten

pinch of paprika

Instructions

STEP 1

Heat the oven to 180C/160C fan/gas 4. Unroll the pastry sheet on its baking parchment. Cut the sheet in half lengthways to create two long rectangles. Squeeze the sausagemeat from its skin into a bowl, then take half and mould into a log across the middle of one of the rectangles. Brush the longer edge of the pastry that's closest to you with a little of the egg. Repeat the process with the remaining filling, pastry and a little more of the beaten egg.

STEP 2

Fold the unglazed edge over the filling on each piece of pastry, then fold the glazed edge over that, pressing gently along the length to seal. Turn the sausage rolls over, tucking the seal underneath, then gently squeeze the pastry around the sausage filling. Use a sharp knife to cut each sausage roll into seven pieces, then lift them, still on the parchment, onto a baking tray. The rolls can now be frozen on the tray. Once solid, put in a freezerproof container and freeze for up to three months.

STEP 3

Brush the top of each sausage roll with the remaining beaten egg and sprinkle with a pinch of paprika and some sea salt. Bake for 25-30 mins (or 40 mins from frozen) until golden brown. Leave to cool for at least 10 mins before eating.

Sweet popcorn

Ingredients

2 tbsp vegetable oil

100g popcorn kernels

250g caster sugar

50g salted butter, cubed

Instructions

STEP 1

Put the oil in a large saucepan with a tight-fitting lid over a medium heat. Toss the popcorn kernels in the oil to coat. Put the lid on, and keep over a medium heat until you hear the first popcorn pop, then turn the heat to medium-low. When you begin to hear lots of popping, give the pan a shake. Continue to shake frequently until the popping stops. Turn off the heat and leave in the pan.

STEP 2

Line a large baking tray with baking parchment. Put the sugar and 60ml water into a medium heavy-based saucepan and bring to the boil. Stir until the sugar has dissolved, then leave over a medium heat, without stirring, for 6-8 mins. It should start to turn into a

golden caramel, swirl it around and add the butter –
stand back as it may spit a little. Stir well until
combined.

STEP 3

Pour the caramel over the popcorn in the pan and stir
immediately to coat the popcorn, being careful not to
touch the hot caramel. Carefully transfer onto the lined
baking tray and press down with the back of a spoon
to spread evenly. Leave to cool for 5 mins, then break
apart and eat.

Beetroot hummus

Ingredients

500g raw beetroot, leaves trimmed to 1 inch, but root left whole

2 x 400g cans chickpeas, drained

juice 2 lemons

1 tbsp ground cumin

yogurt, toasted cumin seeds, mint and crusty bread, to serve

Instructions

STEP 1

Cook the beetroot in a large pan of boiling water with the lid on for 30-40 mins until tender. When they're done, a skewer or knife should go all the way in easily. Drain, then set aside to cool.

STEP 2

Pop on a pair of rubber gloves. Pull off and discard the roots, leaves/stalk and peel of the cooled beetroot. Roughly chop the flesh. Whizz the beetroot, chickpeas, lemon juice, cumin, 2 tsp salt and some pepper. Serve swirled with a little yogurt, some toasted cumin seeds, a little torn mint and some crusty bread.

CHAPTER VI: BEFORE YOU GO, HERE'S A FINAL REMINDER!

In conclusion, managing diet after an ileostomy is crucial for maintaining health and well-being. While it may initially seem daunting, with proper guidance and support from healthcare providers, individuals can navigate dietary changes effectively. Tailoring the diet to suit personal preferences and tolerances, along with staying hydrated and mindful of nutritional needs, can help individuals thrive with an ileostomy. Embracing a balanced approach that includes a variety of foods while being attentive to potential triggers or challenges can lead to a fulfilling and enjoyable dietary experience post-ileostomy surgery.